Social Media and Mental Health
Handbook for Parents and Teachers

BY DR CLAIRE EDWARDS

THE AUTHOR

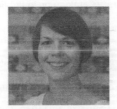

Dr Claire Edwards (BSc (Hons), PG Cert, PsychD, PG Dip)
is a Clinical Psychologist based in London. She first began
working in child and adolescent mental health services in
2001 and has been working as a clinical psychologist since
qualifying in 2008.

Claire has worked with families in a variety of settings,
working with individuals, parents / carers, families, groups
and schools, assessing and treating the mental health
and behavioural difficulties that children and adolescents
present with.

Claire has had a longstanding interest in the broader
factors which impact the lives of young people and their
families and a passion for enhancing family relationships.

Claire is also a parent, so she also has a personal
interest in the wider influences on families and how they
affect relationships.

First published in Great Britain 2018 by Trigger

The Foundation Centre
Navigation House, 48 Millgate, Newark
Nottinghamshire NG24 4TS UK

www.triggerpublishing.com

British Library Cataloguing in Publication Data

A CIP catalogue record for this book is available upon
request from the British Library

ISBN: 978-1-911246-69-5

This book is also available in the following e-Book formats:

MOBI: 978-1-911246-72-5
EPUB: 978-1-911246-70-1
PDF: 978-1-911246-71-8

This book is also available to purchase as a bundle with our
Social Media and Mental Health Handbook for Teens :)
BUNDLE: 978-1-912478-25-5

Claire Edwards has asserted her right under the Copyright,
Design and Patents Act 1988 to be identified
as the author of this work

Cover design and typeset by Fusion Graphic Design Ltd

Printed and bound in Great Britain by Clays Ltd, Elcograf S.p.A

Paper from responsible sources

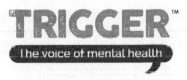

www.triggerpublishing.com

**Thank you for purchasing this book.
You are making an incredible difference.**

Proceeds from all Trigger books go directly to
The Shaw Mind Foundation, a global charity that
focuses entirely on mental health. To find out more
about The Shaw Mind Foundation, visit
www.shawmindfoundation.org

MISSION STATEMENT

*Our goal is to make help and support available for every
single person in society, from all walks of life. We will
never stop offering hope. These are our promises.*

Trigger and The Shaw Mind Foundation

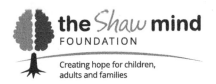

Creating hope for children,
adults and families

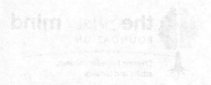

CONTENTS

CONTENTS

INTRODUCTION

The internet is a complex and compelling world – and one that young people today well and truly inhabit. Our children are the first generation to be completely immersed in the digital culture from birth, in a way that we were not. Parents have always faced new challenges and had to adapt to changes in technology – think about the introduction of the television into households. At that time, it was the most powerful communication technology available[1]. But the internet has evolved so rapidly – and become such a large influence across cultures – that we need to carefully consider how to manage it, both for our children and ourselves as parents.

Our children and young people are "digital natives"[2] – they have grown up in this world of the internet and social media. We, on the other hand, are "digital immigrants"[3], born before the advent and rise of digital technologies. This world is, in some ways, foreign to us. Our world views and cultural frames of reference are inherently different; we hold different views about each other and speak different languages. This can create difficulties across the generations. It can also create a lot of fear for parents and carers.

We are learning about the impact of the rapid rise of the internet and social media on young people. This can make navigating our way through the digital landscape as parents a tricky endeavour, and it can be hard to get concrete and clear advice. The research so far hasn't quite caught up with the fast-paced internet, and it can be inconclusive. Raising children can be challenging at the best of times, and this added layer of complexity is one that we need to manage effectively in order to support the physical and emotional development of our children.

The internet has revolutionised the way we communicate and access information. The earliest forms of the internet were developed in the 1960s as a network to link research institutions. By the 1970s, networking technology had improved. By the 1980s, home computers were becoming more readily available and social media more sophisticated. From the 1980s the internet grew beyond just being a research facility, and it began to include a broader community of users. It became more commercial in its activity.

In 1988, Internet Relay Chats and bulletin board systems were first used to enable group communication in discussion forums, as well as one-to-one private communication, and in many ways formed the precursors to social networking as we know it now. One of the biggest changes which had a huge impact on how the internet was used was the shift from web 1.0 to web 2.0. Web 1.0 was content focused – you would go to a website and read its information, but not interact with anyone or change what it said. Web 2.0 is now a communication medium – you can communicate with a global community, change the content of some websites and create online communities.

Web 2.0 has become far more relational now, but was never developed with children in mind. Despite this, one third of internet users are under the age of 18[4]. The speed at which the internet changes is also phenomenal, making it hard to keep up with the latest trends and preferred ways of doing things. Children are growing up with this as an integral part of their lives, whereas we have had to learn to accommodate it. In fact, it's quite likely that your child knows much more about the internet and social media than you do, which sets up an interesting dynamic.

The other major change has been the introduction of smartphones and tablets. Much more portable than laptops and personal computers, these devices can be used anywhere, anytime. They are also often for personal, and not communal, use, which changes how they are viewed and used. In 2016, 82% of adults (classed as 16 years old and over) in Great Britain were using the internet daily or almost daily, and 72% of adults were using mobile or smartphones to access the internet.[5] Even the way we watch television has now changed. With digital television, streaming services and the internet, we can now watch programmes whenever we like. As parents often point out to me, there's no point in banning the television as a consequence anymore, as children can just catch up with their favourite programmes online.

This book comes from a place of positive intentions in supporting parents and carers in somewhat uncharted territory. It is based on my therapeutic work with families, along with research and current recommendations. As with everything, there will be parts of this that will fit for you, and other parts that won't. You will take away what is useful for you and I hope that it will help you think about the most helpful way of managing things in your family.

However, I think it's important to note that managing your child's use of social media has to be seen within the context of how you parent, and your family life more generally. If you do not have the basics in place first, then anything you do to manage difficulties may actually make things worse. Imposing rules and boundaries if your relationship with your child is not positive may only serve to push them further away and increase their retreat into the virtual world. The way we use the internet is relational, and just like the in the way you support your child in order to build positive relationships in the real world, you also want to help them do this in the virtual world.

The process of writing this book has also made me think about my own use of technology and social media. It has made me realise how much I use my smartphone and encouraged me to take a look at the function of social media in my life. It has reinforced the importance of establishing good habits early on in my family, and it's helped me think about how I want to shape my children's use of the internet for now and for the future. Sometimes the best choice is not the easiest one, but as with lots of things in parenting you have to hold on to the hope that the hard work pays off in the future. And as the old adage goes, prevention is better than cure, and it definitely applies in this area. The internet does have some aspects to be wary of, but it also offers many creative opportunities and positive ways to connect with a global community.

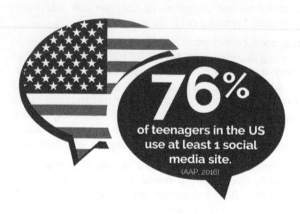

CHAPTER 1

AGES AND STAGES: CHILDREN'S DEVELOPMENT AND THEIR USE OF SOCIAL MEDIA

A child's development is based on a number of things. The nature vs. nurture debate shows that environment, temperament and innate ability all play a part in how children and adolescents develop into adulthood. Much of developmental psychology is based on Western ideas, but it still offers us useful information about child development and how we can help support it – especially now that social media plays such a big role in our lives.

The number of children and teenagers owning mobile phones is steadily increasing, along with their use of social media. Research shows that parents / carers can shape the growth of their child's brain according to the experiences they offer, and hours of screen time will wire the brain in a particular way.[6]

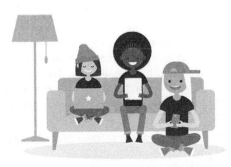

The challenge for you, as parents or carers, is how to incorporate the internet in their lives in a way that *facilitates* their development, rather than hindering it.

So, how does a child's development progress through the age ranges, and how can social media impact their lives – for better or for worse?

BABIES AND TODDLERS

Babies need to develop a secure attachment to their primary caregiver in order to have a secure base from which to explore the world. It gives them a good template for forming relationships with others and helps them communicate their needs.

Babies and toddlers need adults to be both physically and emotionally present with them. They need eye contact, lots of talking to (even when they cannot talk) and reciprocity. And so limiting your own time on devices so that you can be available for them can really help with this.

It also sets up the foundations of your child's relationship with electronic devices as they grow up.

The transition to parenthood can be a very challenging time, and time on technology can be a way of managing this. It can help you find relevant information, share worries with other parents, and get some "me time." But just being with your baby and toddler is so invaluable, and having times that are not interrupted by your mobile phone is crucial.

I know myself how easy it is to get immersed in social media as a way to feel connected with the outside world when you're alone with a small baby. This is absolutely fine, but it's a good idea to try to monitor how much you're doing it, and the message that you may be giving your child.

It may be useful to ban your own use of devices until nap time or at certain points in the day.[7]

DID YOU KNOW?

Research seems to suggest there is little benefit in babies and toddlers under the age of two engaging in media for social and cognitive development. Prior to the age of two, there is no educational value in screen time.[8]

It can be tough, but the reality is that it is better for this age group not to engage in social media. If they do, it's best in moderation. Ideally, they would also do it *with you*, so that it is still interactive.

There are so many benefits to limiting the use of social media and other electronic devices at this stage of your child's life – especially if you turn them off when you say you will. Here's just a few:

- This is the easiest time to limit exposure – and you're setting up good patterns of behaviour for the future.

- It creates time for you both when there are **no distractions.** As you're laying the foundations for language development, making time to just talk and interact with your baby or toddler is vital.

- You have time do things together with your baby that help them focus on a game or task for short periods of time – which is crucial for your relationship and developing their concentration skills.

- You are also helping your child learn how to interact with other adults and children as they develop social skills – all of which can only be done with face-to-face interaction.

- It also limits your baby or toddler's exposure to advertising, which is an important matter for a lot of parents and guardians.

YOUNG CHILDREN (AGED 3 – 5)

Young children are sponges for information. Their physical, emotional, social and psychological development is rapid at this point in their lives. As they venture out into the world, they are exposed to more and more external influences.

Between the ages of three and five, their language develops quickly and they learn how to express themselves. They make meaningful relationships with others. Relationships with their peers become more complex and there is more social pressure.

At this stage their gross and fine motor skills improve too, and they start to achieve physical milestones such as hopping, throwing, riding a bike, holding a pencil and beginning to write.

As your child starts school they will also start to use technology as part of their exploration and education. There are some educational apps that can help your child learn numbers, colours, and writing, but it's best that these are used in addition to – and not instead of – doing things directly with your child to help their learning.

DID YOU KNOW?

Interestingly, there are people who believe that the iPhone is the most effective teaching tool since the invention of chalk and the slate board, and that it can help prepare children for formal learning.[9]

Studies suggest that 55% of 3 to 4-year-olds in the UK now use a tablet, with 16% of them owing their own tablet and 37% using YouTube.[10]

This age group is much more likely to be supervised when using a tablet, although they are often able to navigate the internet by themselves. It's really important to supervise them as much as you can, as they can easily find their way onto unsuitable websites.

MIDDLE CHILDHOOD AND TWEENS

At this stage, your child is fully established in their school life. Peer and academic pressure mounts. You have less influence over what they are exposed to as they spend more time with their friends at school. They will become much more aware of different aspects of their identity, such as gender, and will choose carefully who they play and interact with.

They are learning to understand social rules, develop ideas about what is right and wrong and become increasingly independent. They can now actually read and begin to understand the full content of websites. At this point your child might also have their own mobile phone, particularly if they are doing things like travelling to and from school on their own.

Here's some info about social media use in this age group:[11]

- In the UK in 2016, 32% of 8 to 11-year-olds had their own mobile phone. This number is rising.

- 54% of 5 to 7-year-olds and 73% of 8 to 11-year-olds use YouTube. Around half consider Facebook their main social media profile.

- The preference for mobile phones seems to begin at age 11, with most saying that they would miss their mobile phone the most out of all digital devices if it was taken away.

- The number of children with a social media profile doubles between the age of 10 and 11.

- 11% of 8 to 11-year-olds are checking their social media account more than 10 times a day.

ADOLESCENCE

Adolescence is a huge period of change.

Friends and peer groups become much more important when your child becomes a teenager. They begin to separate from the family more and develop their own independence. The brain is being remodelled, with connections that are no longer used being pruned away. The last part of the brain to be remodelled is the front (the prefrontal cortex), which is involved in problem solving, controlling impulses and thinking about consequences. As a result, teenagers continue to rely more on another part of their brain, the amygdala, which uses emotions, impulses and instinct to make decisions.

This, combined with an influx of hormones, can make your teenager's behaviour challenging. They might want to take more risks. They're likely to become much more interested in sex.

DID YOU KNOW?

By age 12, half of all children in the UK have a social media profile.[12]

In 2011, almost half of 11 to 16-year-olds said it was easier to be themselves online than face to face.[13]

Adolescents often want to connect more with their peers, and social media is an instant way to reach people. This has pros and cons, especially when there's less problem solving and more impulsivity going on! There's a higher risk of conflict and teens comparing themselves to one another, but social media can also be a nice way to create new relationships and find a different kind of support network.

We are all social beings in our own way, and the internet is just an extension of this.

Here are some more interesting stats from the UK:[14]

- 79% of 12 to 15-year-olds have their own mobile phone.

- 87% of this age group use YouTube and 52% consider Facebook as their main social media profile.

- A staggering 74% of adolescents have a social media profile by the age of 13.

- Research shows that many young people use social media in the evening, with some targeting their posts for this time as they are more likely to get responses from their peers.

- 38% of 11 to 15-year-olds use social media at 8.15pm, 15% at 9.00pm, and 2% at midnight. Given the impact that exposure to screens has on sleep, this is clearly not an encouraging trend.

This age group is beginning to develop their "critical understanding" of their media environment. They are becoming more able to **understand, question and manage information** so that they can use the internet effectively.

DID YOU KNOW?

Interestingly, research suggests that whether or not a teenager questions information depends on its context:

- Often teens will actively question information if it is for homework or something important, but not for entertainment.

- As young people try harder and harder to fit in and their peers become more influential in their lives, they are less likely to challenge information that they would have done previously.

- 27% of 12 to 15-year-olds said that if they googled a website they would trust it.[15]

CHAPTER 2

WHAT'S OUT THERE?

In 2016, 23% of children aged 8–11 and 72% of children aged 12–15 in the UK had a social media profile. That's a big number for such young people.

Not only that, but this number doubled to 21–43% for children who are 10 and 11 years old, and increased to 50–74% between 12 and 13-year-olds.[16]

When you consider that children and young people are using social media in the evening (a tenth of 11 to 15-year-olds are still communicating via social media at 10.00pm[17]) and using likes and shares as a form of social currency, these websites are having a huge impact on young people in terms of their sleeping habits and identity formation.

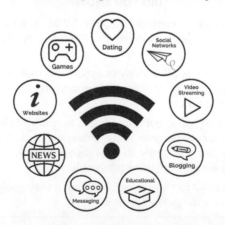

While the internet is fast-paced and will therefore have inevitably moved on even since this book was published, it is important to have some knowledge about what is on the internet and how your child(ren) might be accessing it. Below are some of the most popular types of app, social networking site or websites accessed by children and young people.

DEVICES

The internet can be accessed through a variety of devices. Initially you could only access the internet through desktop computers and laptops, but this has now evolved to include games consoles, mobile phones, tablets and smart televisions. This has led to some unique challenges in managing internet and social media use within the family. When the internet was first used by young people at home, the advice was to leave the computer in a public area so that parents / carers could monitor its usage. The difficulty now is that the internet is used on personal and portable devices, which are often used outside of the family home or in private areas such as bedrooms. This makes effective monitoring a much more challenging task for parents, carers, teachers or guardians, especially when keeping an eye on content and managing boundaries around frequency and amount of internet use.

In 2016, tablets – followed by mobile phones – were the most popular devices for children and young people to access the internet. The numbers of children who own mobile phones are on the increase.[18]

DID YOU KNOW?

Young people show a preference for accessing the internet using mobile phones at 11 years of age, and boys are more likely to own a games console which they can also use to access the internet.[19]

TIPS FOR MANAGING INTERNET USAGE ON YOUR CHILDREN AND FAMILY'S DEVICES

For younger children:

- For younger kids, use search engines like www.swiggle.org.uk/ and www.kids-search.com/ and set your homepage to a child friendly website, such as CBeebies.

- Set up user accounts with passwords on your computer for each child, which only allow them to use appropriate websites.

- Have a family email address to use for signing up for apps.

- Make sure passwords are strong and never given to anyone else.

For teens and adolescents:

- Be on the lookout for changes in your child's behaviour and mood which might indicate that something concerning is happening (online or offline).

- Be worried if your child has new possessions or money and you don't know where they have come from.

- Have an open and honest discussion with them about the risks and dangers associated with internet and social media use (more on this in "The Darker Side of the Internet" chapter).

For the family:

- Where possible, use the internet together at home and encourage your family to use their devices together in communal family areas, such as the living room.

- Have a central charging area where all phones can charge overnight
- Think about your own use – what are you modelling for your children in terms of your internet habits?
- Set up a family internet plan – see the "Managing Social Media Use and Building a Plan" chapter!

WHAT TYPES OF SOCIAL MEDIA, APPS AND WEBSITES ARE MOST POPULAR WITH CHILDREN AND YOUNG PEOPLE?

Video Streaming Sites

Video streaming sites and apps – the most notable, at present, being YouTube – are incredibly popular right now, especially among children, adolescents and young people. They can be a mine of information, entertainment and knowledge, and can open up whole new worlds for people, without them ever having to leave their homes.

EXAMPLE:

YouTube

YouTube is a video sharing website that allows users to upload videos of their own and watch videos posted by other users across the globe. Their mission, "to give everyone a voice and show them the world," is certainly well realised. The platform is used by individuals who can set up their own accounts for free. They can post videos, watch other videos without signing up for an account, and develop a huge online following. Businesses also use the app in order to advertise and promote themselves.

YouTube hosts millions of videos that show a wide range of content – anything from amateur films to vlogging (a video form of "blogging" or "web logging", a way of sharing experiences, observations, and opinions), music videos, and instructional videos. Anyone who has a free YouTube account can then write comments about the videos, and users can like or dislike what they see. Users open themselves up to both positive and negative feedback and encourage their "fans" to subscribe to their channel.

YouTube was acquired by Google in 2006 and as a result offers revenue sharing for advertisement clicks, so some users have been able to make money from posting their videos. Some of the young people I have worked with aspire to be professional YouTubers.

DID YOU KNOW?

Older children prefer using YouTube to watching content on the TV.

In a report by Ofcom, when asked whether they prefer watching YouTube or watching TV programmes on a TV set, 42% of 8 to 11-year-olds and 41% of 12 to 15-year-olds said they were much more likely to opt for YouTube.

This may be related to the fact that when asked about TV, around one in four 8 to 11-year-old, and almost a third of 12 to 15-year-olds complained that there are not enough programmes that they like on the TV.

YouTube is an increasingly important content destination. It is popular across all ages, particularly among older children. As of 2017, 37% of children aged 3–4, 54% of children aged 5–7, 73% of those aged 8–11 and 87% of 12 to 15-year-olds use the YouTube website or app.

The content children like to watch on YouTube differs by age. Younger children (3–7) are most likely to watch TV programmes, films, cartoons, mini-movies, animations or songs, and parents say that this is their child's favourite type of YouTube content.

As children get older, they tend to prefer watching music videos, funny videos or pranks, and content posted by "vloggers". Research suggests that vloggers in particular are an important source of teen orientated content.

The website contains YouTube's policies on community guidelines, staying safe and reporting and enforcement. They clearly state what is and isn't acceptable in terms of content and how to report inappropriate content or activity. But the challenge for YouTube – along with other social media sites – is the speed at which they can detect and remove inappropriate content or activity, given the vast amount of material uploaded daily and comments made.

CONCERNS

There are some significant risks and potential dangers associated with video streaming sites. These include:

- The potential for young children to stumble across sexual or age-inappropriate content. Parents and carers are often concerned that their young children will easily be able to stumble upon this kind of material, even when the child isn't actively searching for it.

- The risk of being exposed to disturbing, violent or traumatising material.

- Copyright infringement.

- The prevalence of revenge porn.

- "Related content" suggestions, leading children towards unwanted videos without them realising.

- Children becoming exposed to commercial advertising.

- Privacy issues, lack of understanding of terms and conditions, and difficulties in monitoring use.

TIPS FOR MANAGING YOUR CHILD'S USE OF VIDEO STREAMING APPS:

- Download YouTube Kids for younger children.

- Take the time to read through the app's terms and conditions thoroughly.

- Check the minimum age restrictions and make sure your child is not using any app or website while underage.

- Take advantage of the parental controls on video apps and websites, if there are any. On YouTube, for example, you can go to settings, tick "safe search filtering" and tick "strict". Check Google or the site's FAQ page to find out how to navigate this on other sites.

- Make sure, where possible, that you regularly review what your child is accessing, especially younger children.

- For teens and adolescents, make sure to discuss their use of YouTube and other video streaming apps regularly, advising them to be careful of potential harmful material.

- Build the use of video streaming apps into a social media / internet plan or agreement, if you choose to make one.

Social Networking Sites

There is a huge array of social networking apps, websites and platforms that allow users to set up their own public or private profile, on which they can share photos, information, and updates about their day-to-day lives. Social networking sites are a fantastic way of staying in touch with friends, and they're especially useful for keeping in contact with people who live a long way away. They're also great for hosting and sharing news stories.

EXAMPLE:

Facebook

Facebook is a popular social media website developed by Mark Zuckerberg when he was a student at Harvard University. In order to use it you need to set up a profile, which asks for information about you. "Friends" are then added to your page via requests, which you can accept or deny. You can post status updates, upload photos and videos, and comment and like other people's statuses.

Businesses can create pages and use them to promote themselves, using a basic free page or paying to advertise services. People can also use the platform to create groups and event pages.

Users can set privacy settings so that only "friends" can see their entire page and have access to their photos, or allow open access so that anyone is able to view it.

DID YOU KNOW?

Facebook has an enormous following. Ofcom (2016) reported that 43% of 8 to 11-year-olds 12 to 15-year-olds (52%) were most likely to consider Facebook their main social media profile. In October 2012, Facebook had one billion monthly users, and in July 2017 it announced it had doubled to two billion monthly users[20]. That's over a quarter of the world's population using Facebook!

A rapid rise in user numbers is the reason for ongoing concerns about how Facebook is able to monitor and moderate the content posted on its site. In the past there have been some difficulties in getting distressing or offensive content taken down from the platform. Some recent shocking examples of this include footage from the US; one video involved a 14-year-old live streaming her own suicide, while another showed a man shooting and killing an elderly man. Facebook announced in May 2017 that they were employing an additional 3,000 workers to moderate content.

In recent years, Facebook has also come under considerable pressure and criticism for its handling of users' private data.

Twitter

Launched in 2006, Twitter is a website that enables users to publish short messages ("tweets") of up to 280 characters. Users "follow" other users (and therefore become "followers"), in order to see these updates. Unless a user changes their privacy settings, anyone can follow a particular person's profile. Users can retweet or quote other people and leave their own tweets in reply. Twitter is widely used by individuals, but companies and organisations also use it for promotional and customer service purposes. Many people use it as a way to keep up to date with national and international news accounts, and real-time events are often played out on Twitter.

Twitter is a popular way for people to connect with others. Many celebrities and politicians have Twitter accounts with millions of followers. Users regularly use hashtags on Twitter in order to be found online more easily, to organise content and be linked into themes. Popular topics are described as "trending" when a large number of people are all tweeting about the same thing at the same time, often using the same hashtag.

CONCERNS

Social networking sites come with their own risks and potential dangers. These include:

- People's data being shared without their consent, even by verified apps

- Users accepting terms and conditions without reading them and understanding what they're agreeing to.

- Oversharing of personal and private information without thought for the consequences.

- Trolling, where certain people are targeted and attacked either by strangers or people they know.

- "Witch hunting", in which people are subjected to public shaming or harassment for something they may or may not have done.

- "Fake news" – sharing of information that is not verified, has no source, or is simply untrue.

- People sharing fake news or fake accusations without corroboration.

- People stealing photographs or other people's information without consent.

- "Hacking" – someone using someone else's profile to ruin their reputation or access their private data.

- Targeted advertising.

- Cyberbullying.

TIPS FOR SAFELY MANAGING YOUR CHILD'S USE OF SOCIAL MEDIA NETWORKING SITES:

- Make an agreement with your teenager or adolescent as to whether you can follow their profile and keep an eye on their usage.

- Check the minimum age restriction and make sure that your child is not underage.

- Discuss with them the dangers of sharing too much of their personal or private information (there is more information on this in later chapters).

- Ensure they don't leave their Facebook or other account logged in so other people can access it.

- Set up passwords on devices so that they can't be accessed if left unattended.

- Tell them to check their privacy settings and make sure that only people they know can see their photos, information and updates.

- Encourage them to, where possible, set up their settings so that they can decide what photos they are tagged in.

- Remind your teens that whatever they put online affects their safety and online reputation. Tell them to **think twice** and **carefully consider** everything they post before they post it.

- Have a regular conversation with your child to make sure they feel safe and address any concerns they might have.

- Make sure they know how to report concerns and block inappropriate content. Sites should have FAQ pages that will provide you with this information.

- For advice on Facebook hacking, visit www.facebook.com/hacked.

Photo Apps and Websites

Apps and platforms on which people can post photos of themselves, their friends and are lives are incredibly popular, especially among children and young people. Some of the most popular types of photos that people post on these apps are "selfies", which are photos that individuals take of themselves.

EXAMPLE:

Instagram

Instagram is a website designed for posting and sharing photos with friends via an app on your smartphone or device. There are ways to enhance, edit and alter photos, such as using filters to make them appear brighter or more aged, like an old Polaroid photo, for instance. Instagram is a great tool for fostering creativity and inspiring budding photographers and filmmakers. Friends can tag each other in their photos and, just like with Twitter, they can use hashtags in order to be found more easily online. Just like on Twitter, you gather "followers" on Instagram, and gathering a higher following can become very important to some people. Interestingly, Instagram was acquired by Facebook in 2012, along with other social media apps and platforms.

DID YOU KNOW?

The Children's Commissioner[21] tested young people's understanding of the terms and conditions of Instagram. 56% of 12 to 15-year-olds and 43% of 8 to 11-year-olds in 2017 had an Instagram account, so it is important to explore young people's understanding of their rights in relation to social media. The terms and conditions for use were 17 pages long, 5,000 words in length and used sentence structure that only a postgraduate could be expected to understand!

The young people involved begged to stop when they had only got through half the text, because they felt that they couldn't understand it. As with most social media sites, the report highlights that young people must understand that "you waive fundamental privacy; the app could track you even when not in use; your personal data could be bought and sold; the terms could change at any time without notice, and the app could terminate your account as its sole discretion."

Ofcom asked a law firm to write the terms and conditions in a simpler way which the young people could engage with and understand. Their ideas about using Instagram changed once they were more informed and understood their rights. One young person even deleted their account as a result.

CONCERNS

Understandably, any platform that allows children and young people to share photos publicly can cause unease for parents and carers. Some worries include:

- Instagram and similar apps can result in a lack of privacy.

- Children and young people are often unaware of their personal rights and rules around copyright.

- Users can often have their photos stolen and used elsewhere online without their knowledge or consent.

- Instagram and other photo apps may contribute to people feeling FOMO – a fear of missing out.

- Photo editing apps and software can lead children and young people to believe that the "perfect" or "ideal" images they see online are real, and therefore they will feel inadequate and self-conscious as a result.

TIPS FOR SAFELY MANAGING YOUR CHILD'S USE OF SOCIAL MEDIA NETWORKING SITES:

- Make sure that your child understands the risks of using photo apps, such as a lack of privacy.

- Have a discussion with them about their need to edit their photos if they feel the need to do so.

- Make them aware of the option to make their photos private rather than public.

- Remind them that if their profile is public, their teachers, friends, family and future employers can see their posts – especially as they can leave a digital footprint even when deleted.

- Point out that they can use the blocking and reporting functions if they are attacked online or made to feel uncomfortable.

- Tell them to bear in mind that a lot of photos online are edited, and therefore they often present a false representation of reality.

- Have a wider discussion with them about their confidence, self-esteem and body image if you're worried that their mental health is being affected.

Messaging Apps

There are a huge variety of messaging apps available for free, and they are particularly popular with children and young people. For teenagers especially, staying in touch with friends is incredibly important, and messaging apps provide a free and fun way to do so.

EXAMPLES:

Snapchat

Snapchat is a photo or video sharing app, on which any content that is shared is time sensitive. A picture can only be viewed for a few seconds before it disappears. If a screenshot is taken of the image, then the user is alerted. Users can now also add to their "stories", feeds that last for just 24 hours before disappearing. Some people aspire to get the longest Snapchat streak, which is when users send each other direct snaps without missing a day. Snapchat streaks can become quite addictive because users are "rewarded" with emojis (small illustrative icons often used in text and online messaging) when they reach certain milestones.

There has been recent controversy around this app, which added another feature – Snap Maps – of which many users were unaware. This is a feature which enables users to see exactly where their friends are and what they are doing. You can also view videos and / or photos of strangers who are posting from popular events or locations. The app needs to be changed to "ghost mode" in order for data not to be shared. Many parents, carers and even children were, understandably, upset because they hadn't been made aware of this breach of privacy, one which holds significant safety risks for young people.

WhatsApp

WhatsApp is an instant messaging service which can be used on smartphones, tablets and desktops. It works a little bit like text messaging. There's no cost to message friends, as it uses an internet connection. You can use it for one-on-one conversations or set up a group, and it can be used to share messages, images, and videos. You can also use voice message and make telephone calls. Users can update their status to let other users know whether or not they are available.

WhatsApp was acquired by Facebook in 2014. It attracted controversy in 2016 when it announced that it would start sharing account information with Facebook, and users had to ensure their privacy settings did not consent to this if they didn't want it to happen.

CONCERNS

While the opportunity to easily message friends and family is a positive thing, parents and guardians do have some worries about messaging apps, including the following:

- The prevalence of cyberbullying on messaging apps, especially on Snapchat, where offensive posts can disappear.
- The potential for data breaches and risks.
- Location services making children and young people easy to locate and track down.
- The risk of grooming and online child sexual exploitation.

TIPS FOR MANAGING YOUR CHILD'S USE OF MESSAGING APPS:

- Help them check their privacy settings.
- Have a conversation with them about cyberbullying and grooming (more on this in "The Darker Side of the Internet" chapter).
- Set clear boundaries within the household regarding time spent on messaging apps.
- Check or monitor their online conduct and who they're talking to.

Blogging Sites

While the sharing of visual content such as videos and photos becomes ever more popular, there are still a lot of children and young people who write and create blogs ("web logs", writing that discusses a wide range of topics, including food, fandoms, hobbies, lifestyle, gaming and beauty).

There are many blog hosting sites out there that allow users to host their blogs for free.

Blogging is a brilliant way for budding young writers, journalists, and photographers to build on their skills and foster their creativity.

EXAMPLE:

Tumblr

Tumblr is a social networking and microblogging (small blogs consisting of a few sentences) site. Users have a "dashboard" which allows them to see a live feed of the blogs they follow, which they can like, comment on and repost. Users can also connect their account to other sites such as Facebook and Twitter, so posting on Tumblr would then automatically send a tweet and / or Facebook post. It was set up in 2007 and acquired by Yahoo in 2013.

Tumblr has been criticised for its adult content (most notably pornography) and also for hosting content glorifying or depicting self-harm, suicide, and eating disorders. In 2012, Tumblr changed its policy and banned content that promoted these issues with links to support organisations provided.

CONCERNS

- The risk of young people accessing inappropriate content, such as pornography, misogyny, discrimination, racism, or posts glamorising self-harm and eating disorders.

- Exposure to negative comments and trolling.

- Lack of privacy or risk of oversharing information.

> ### TIPS FOR MONITORING YOUR CHILD'S USE OF BLOGGING SITES:
>
> - Have a conversation about the above concerns and warn them about potential harmful content.
> - Check to see if there are any parental controls you can apply to the site.
> - Discuss with them the importance of not oversharing or giving out private information.

Online Gaming

The online gaming world is incredibly big and diverse. An activity that is available on a variety of devices and consoles, online gaming allows players to connect through the internet and converse with each other through headphones while playing. It is a huge industry which garners massive followings, hosts worldwide events and conventions, and produces millions of pounds worth of merchandising. It is particularly popular with - but not limited to - young boys.

Examples of popular consoles include:

- Xbox
- Nintendo
- PlayStation
- Desktop computers (PCs)

Examples of popular games include:

- World of Warcraft (roleplaying)
- Minecraft
- Halo
- Destiny
- Grand Theft Auto
- Fortnite

DID YOU KNOW?

It is estimated that 5% of young people in The Netherlands are addicted to online gaming.[22]

Research at the University of Amsterdam used the following nine criteria[23] (taken from the internet gaming disorder scale from the Diagnostic and Statistical Manual of Mental Disorders (DSM–5)[24]) to assess whether young people were addicted:

- Preoccupation: spending substantial amounts of time thinking about gaming.

- Tolerance: needing to spend an increasing amount of time to feel the desired effect (excitement, etc.).

- Withdrawal: feeling restless, irritated, angry, frustrated, anxious or sad when unable play games.

- Persistence: unsuccessful attempts to stop, control or reduce the amount of the time spent gaming.

- Escape: using gaming to relieve negative mood states.

- Problems: ongoing usage despite being aware of negative consequences.

- Deception: lying or covering up the extent of usage.

- Displacement: reduced social or recreational activities as a result of continued gaming.

- Conflict: losing or nearly losing an important relationship or opportunity.[25]

In this study, the average teenager was found to spend three hours on social media platforms and another three hours playing computer games per day. The Netherlands was the first European country to get broadband internet, so it is likely that other countries will follow suit with these trends. And that's worrying!

CONCERNS

With the prevalence of online gaming within the child and adolescent community comes some real worries for parents and guardians.

- Addiction to gaming, as above.

- Desensitisation, especially to violent or misogynistic content.

- Isolation and reduced amount of time socialising in the real world.

- Lack of physical exercise and movement.

- A decline in educational performance or slipping of grades.

- Underage children accessing age-restricted games.

- Children talking to strangers online who might potentially exploit them.

- Spending money on credits / features to use in games.

- Impact on sleep – not only are screens and exciting games over-stimulating, making going to sleep difficult, there is always someone to play with in a global community across different time zones.

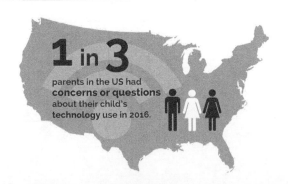

1 in **3** parents in the US had **concerns or questions** about their child's technology use in 2016.

TIPS FOR MANAGING YOUR CHILD'S USE OF ONLINE GAMES:

- Restrict gaming time to certain hours of the day, and for a certain number of hours per day or week.

- No screen time preferably two hours before bedtime.

- Implement an agreed curfew and stick to it.

- Make sure that your child is not playing any games for which they are underage.

- Monitor who they talk to online and ensure that they're not conversing with strangers.

- Apply parental controls on your younger children's devices.

CHAPTER 3

THE POSITIVES OF SOCIAL MEDIA

The internet is a vibrant place, full of creativity and energy. It provides us all with instant access to a wealth of information and a network of support that can extend around the world. We are social beings, and the internet can be a fantastic tool to facilitate positive social interaction.

But as a parent or carer, you are likely to be wary. And when your child reaches a certain age – for instance, when they are about to enter secondary school or when their friends start getting their own smartphones – you might find yourself conflicted as to whether or not you should allow your child to get their own device too. There is likely to be significant pressure and you might be unsure what to do for the best.

It's worth bearing in mind that while the online world can be a scary, confusing place at times, it can also be a real force for good for your child. As with most things, it's a mixed picture – a study in 2014 suggested that social media can "enhance belonging, psychosocial wellbeing, and identity development, while at the same time exposing young people to potential negative outcomes."[26]

There is no right or wrong answer. It's all about weighing up the pros and cons for you, your child, and your family. We will discuss the risks and potential dangers of social media, but it's important to recognise all the ways that social media and the internet can enrich your child's life, so that you can make a balanced decision.

So, if you're feeling worried about your child using social media and you're unsure how it can enhance their lives, here are some positives for you to consider!

1. Social media can positively impact some young people's mental health. It has been known to:

- Decrease loneliness and depression.

- Enhance self-esteem and confidence through positive feedback on profiles feel-good posts, community involvement, body positivity and peer validation.[27]

- Help young people experiment with self-identity and self-expression in a safe and positive way.[28]

- Help children feel supported and part of a wider group or network.

- Provide opportunities for young people with mental health difficulties to self-disclose and discuss their symptoms and experiences online in a supportive community.

2. The internet can help children build their social network:

- Some children who are shy or struggle with social anxiety may find talking online more comfortable than face-to-face.

- It gives them a way to stay connected to others, even during times that are difficult for them.

3. Young people can find helpful and useful information online:

- Social media can also provide children and young people with information about their world.

- They can access support lines, advice pages and chat forums hosted by charities and other organisations designed to support young people.

4. The internet can be a great source of knowledge and can help children with their education:

- It can provide access to educational apps and websites.

- It can spark the imagination and help children and teenagers enjoy learning, where they might otherwise struggle in school.

- As long as apps and websites are an add-on to – and not a substitution for – face-to-face interaction and learning, there's no reason why they can't be used in moderation.

- Children and adolescents are sponges for information, and the internet can offer a huge amount of that!

- Using the internet can also give young people control over how they access information, as they seek out websites that fit with their learning style and help to engage them.

5. The internet facilitates and sparks creativity both online and offline:

- It provides children and young people with ideas about which activities to enjoy in their spare time.

- Platforms such as YouTube and other websites help them discover, develop and nurture new practical skills.

- Websites, forums, blogs, vlogging sites and video streaming apps provide a platform for young people to create and share content.

DID YOU KNOW?

30% of 12 to 15-year-olds who use the internet have signed petitions or shared / talked about the news on social media and engaged in civic participation.[29]

Some social media can be incredibly inspiring for young people. There are a whole host of teenagers who have used the power of social media for good, such as challenging global companies, promoting equality, raising awareness, and making change at a staggering level.

CHAPTER 4

THE DARKER SIDE OF THE INTERNET

Some people might prefer not to acknowledge the darker side of the internet. But in order to keep your child safe, both you and your child need to understand some of the more dangerous aspects of the online world. It's important for everyone to recognise the risks and dangers of using computers and social media – not so that you run away scared, but so that your child can continue to use it (if they wish to), with the right knowledge. That way, you can feel reassured that they know how to navigate the digital landscape safely – and you know what to look out for if you suspect that something's wrong.

Listed below are some of the darker aspects of the internet and social media, with some tips and pointers of what to consider when your child is active online.

CYBERBULLYING (OR ONLINE BULLYING)

Cyberbullying is the same as any other form of bullying; the difference here is that it happens online or via a mobile phone instead. The added complexity of it is that the internet can be an anonymous space, so people will feel free to write things that they would not feel able to say face-to-face. This can lead to very malicious content, often without comeback for the bully or bullies.

At its most serious level, cyberbullying has been linked to anxiety, depression, self-harm and suicide in young people and adults. It can have devastating effects.

Examples of cyberbullying include:

- Posting a nasty comment on a profile / photo
- Sending a horrible or abusive private message
- Bullying people on an online game
- Humiliation
- Wrongfully reporting profiles
- Spreading rumours about people online
- Sharing someone's personal information against their will
- Sharing photos or videos of people that they don't like
- Cropping people out of photos or not including someone in a chat
- Pressuring someone into doing something they don't want to do, such as posting sexually explicit photos
- Impersonating someone else online to get them in trouble or ruin their reputation
- Hacking someone else's account in order to do them harm
- Creating malicious websites in order to target people

Why is cyberbullying so dangerous?

Whereas in the real world, where people can "escape" or "hide" from bullying outside of school or at home, it is a lot more difficult to step away from cyberbullying. The virtual world can be accessed anytime, anywhere, and often there's no respite.

The added element of anonymity and the lack of perceived "authority" online means that people can make themselves untraceable, creating anonymous accounts and sending messages without a second thought about the consequences.

The fact that people can't see the immediate effects of cyberbullying right in front of them also often means that people will take bullying a lot further online than they would in real life. On the internet and on social media there's a removed sense of reality, and therefore some people don't hold on to their responsibility to behave in a compassionate way.

Interestingly – and perhaps worryingly – young people say that the internet is the one area of their lives that they do not feel has clear expectations or standards of behaviour that they should stick to.[30]

Certain apps – such as Sarahah, Sayat.me and other messaging platforms which enable young people to make anonymous accounts – have been dubbed "breeding grounds" for hatred and suicide. As this is inconsistent with Google and Apple's policies against harassment, in recent years there have been petitions for these companies to remove such apps from their online stores and change their guidelines.[31] However, new apps are being built all the time, and so it's up to you and your child to stay proactive and vigilant.

DID YOU KNOW?

Cyberbullying is one of the biggest challenges to young people online, with one study showing that 17% of 12 to 20-year-olds in the UK in 2017 had reported experiencing cyberbullying, based on their own definition.[32]

The same study found that:

- Some young people delete their social media profile or stop using social media as a result of cyberbullying.

- Some went on to develop mental health difficulties because of it.

- 71% of young people felt that social media networks were not doing enough to prevent cyberbullying.

- Sadly, 23% felt that cyberbullying was just a part of growing up.

Is my child being cyberbullied?

If you think your child might be being cyberbullied, but you are unsure, here are some of the signs to look out for:

- A dramatic change in behaviour

- A decrease – or, on the other hand, an increase – in the amount of time they spend on social media or computers

- Appearing more distressed, upset, jumpy or angry than is normal, especially after using the internet or their phone

- An unwillingness to go to school

- Secrecy about their online activity and / or avoidance of discussion about social media [33]

- Eating or sleeping less

Managing cyberbullying

In a similar way to "playground" bullying, cyberbullying is often very difficult to control, though there are lots of organisations and schemes that tackle this ever-growing problem. For example, the Stop, Speak, Support campaign – which was launched in the UK in 2017 – and talks about "when the banter turns bad". It recommends that young people should "Stop" (do not share or like negative comments and check the community guidelines), "Speak" (talk to a trusted adult, use the report button on the site, and / or talk to a Childline) and "Support" – (send a supportive message to the person being bullied, spend some time with them, and encourage them to talk with an adult).

But there are things that you can do, as a parent, teacher, or guardian, to help young people who are at risk of online bullying.

Reassuring your child that you are there to talk to about online bullying will really help. Always discuss cyberbullying with your child BEFORE you suspect anything bad is happening, as well as during. Tell them what to look out for and advise them to be vigilant. Reassure them that they can talk to you as soon as they have any growing concerns about themselves or possibly their friends.

If you suspect that your child might be getting bullied online, broach the subject with them, without forcing them to say anything they don't wish to say. They may be fearful that you'll ban them from social media, so make it clear that you don't intend to take away their device(s), but it will help for you to fully understand what is going on.

TIPS

In order to reduce the risk of your child being cyberbullied, you can try the following things:

- Find out what apps, websites and games they're using and what risks each of these might pose to your child.

- Use safety filters and controls on their devices, ensuring that privacy settings are set on social media accounts.[34]

- Teach them to be social media savvy and think about how the content they put out might attract bullying behaviour.

- Remind them to set strong passwords and never to share them, even with their best friends.

What should I do if I find out that my child is being cyberbullied?

- Advise them not to respond to the bullies online.

- Tell them to block bullies where possible to do so.

- Check the community guidelines and report messages on the app if possible.

- Tell them to keep a record and log the bullying activity. If necessary, report the abuse to the school or the police.

- Encourage your child to spend less time online and more time on other activities and face-to-face interactions with their friends.

DO NOT

- Get angry that they didn't tell you sooner. Admitting to being bullied can be very difficult for a child.

- Ban them from using social media altogether, as some children will see this as punishment.

What should I do if I find out my child has been cyberbullying others?

- Try to explore what might be happening in your child's life so that you can understand their motives. Try to also see it as an opportunity for learning. Perhaps they are distressed about something in an area of their life. Have they been on the receiving end of bullying online or offline?

- Help them to develop their empathy and understand what it might be like for the person they have been cyberbullying.

- Help them consider how they might go about repairing the relationship or acknowledging the impact that they have had. Can they send a message / email / text to apologise and offer some sort of explanation?

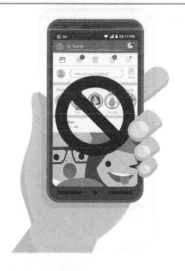

FOMO (FEAR OF MISSING OUT)

This is a growing phenomenon among young people and even adults. Essentially, FOMO (fear of missing out) is that feeling that a person gets when they're worried that other people are enjoying fun events or gatherings when that person can't or isn't there to enjoy it too. This gives them the feeling that they might be "missing out" on life, and this can have a significant impact on a person's mental health, causing anxiety and feelings of personal inadequacy.

FOMO can cause children and young people to spend longer and longer periods of time online – sometimes well into the night – in order to feel as though they're not missing out on an important conversation. Research is limited, but one study reported that young people, particularly males, showed high levels of FOMO. Those who had high levels of FOMO also scored lower levels of life satisfaction and positive mood, and were more likely to use social media before sleep, on waking and during mealtimes and lectures.[35]

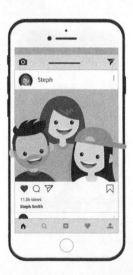

GROOMING AND ONLINE CHILD
SEXUAL EXPLOITATION

It is a sad and unfortunate reality that sexual abuse and grooming happens online, and it is a very real risk all over the world. But by making yourself and your child aware of these dangers, you can help protect them and teach them how to keep themselves safe.

What is grooming and online child sexual exploitation?

Online "grooming" is when someone makes an emotional connection with a child in order to misuse that trust to exploit them. Groomers will often show the child great kindness, compliment them, show them support, offer them help and / or gain their trust. They might also encourage them to move away from, or distrust, their friends, to make them feel like the groomer is the only person they can turn to. The groomer may or may not be known to the child or young person. Online they can easily conceal their identity and pretend to be the same age as the child when they are online, making certain requests seem less odd. The danger is that a lot of children are not aware that this kind of activity takes place, and therefore they are vulnerable to lies and exploitation. The process is subtle. When online, groomers can gather lots of information about a child by looking at things like their social media profile and the information they share about themselves. Groomers may seek out signs of insecurity, low self esteem or neediness[36].

Children, adolescents and teens are particularly vulnerable to grooming, especially since many of them are unaware that this kind of activity takes place. Sexual abuse can happen online, but often the groomer will build up the child's trust and then request to meet them in person.

As outlined by the NSPCC, online child sexual exploitation involves a young person being persuaded to:

- Post sexually explicit images of themselves

- Take part in sexual activities using a camera (webcam, mobile phone), or

- Have sexual conversations online[37].

Once an abuser has an image, they can then use it to further coerce a young person into doing more and more dangerous things, threatening to send the image to family or friends if they do not agree.

How can I help prevent my child from being groomed?

- Warn them of the dangers and signs to look out for.

- Encourage your child to keep their personal information private and help them put privacy settings into place.

- Teach them the dangers of talking to strangers and how adults can pose as children.

- Remind them that if someone they don't know is being nice to them, it doesn't mean they're trustworthy.

- Warn them never to share sexually explicit photos with anyone and explain to them the risks and the consequences.

- Help them develop their confidence so that they are less vulnerable to being targeted.

DID YOU KNOW?

- In 2016, 5% of 12 to 15-year-olds in the UK had sent a picture or video of themselves to someone they had only met online.

- 4% had sent personal information (such as name and address)[38].

Although this could be entirely innocent, it has the potential to make young people incredibly vulnerable, and often they might not realise the risk they are taking.

What should I do if I'm worried that my child is being groomed / abused?

- Broach the subject delicately and reassure them that you're there to keep them safe.

- Remind them that they will not get in trouble for anything that's happened / is happening. Remember, they may have been threatened with something if they tell anyone, which will make it very challenging for them to disclose.

- If they confirm or suspect that they're being groomed, consider using local or national organisations (such as Childline or the Child Exploitation and Online Protection Command) who can help support you and assist you with reporting the abuse.

DO NOT:

- Push them into a conversation if they appear uncomfortable.

- Make them feel judged, ashamed or in any way to blame for what has happened.

EXPOSURE TO DISTURBING, INAPPROPRIATE OR TRAUMATISING CONTENT

It is no secret that there is a very real risk of children and young people accidentally stumbling upon unpleasant content, such as pornography, sexually explicit material, and websites promoting self-harm, eating disorders and other dangerous behaviours. You don't have to search too deeply to find pictures and videos of self-harm or websites promoting eating disorders (for example pro ana). And because it is so easy to be lead, unwittingly, from websites that offer a safe spaces, supportive communities and help with recovery and onto something potentially dangerous instead, there is no wonder that some parents and guardians feel worried and helpless.

The key is how these sites are monitored when easily accessible by young people.

TIPS

- For younger kids, use search engines like www.swiggle.org.uk/ and www.kids-search.com/ and set your homepage to a child friendly website, such as CBeebies.

- Set up user accounts with passwords on your computer for each child, which only allows them to use appropriate websites.

- Set up parental controls where possible on websites and apps.

- For teens and adolescents, have a frank and honest discussion with them about what they might stumble across, and warn them about the types of material that they should avoid online.

"SEXTING" AND REVENGE PORN

"Revenge porn" is the term used to describe when someone takes naked or sexually explicit footage or photos of another person and shares them online without that person's consent. The person may or may not have consented to the images being taken in the first place.

In 2015, the UK brought in a law that made "revenge porn" illegal.

With the rise of "sexting", it's important that your child understands the risks of sending such private material to others, even to those they trust. Revenge porn has been known to occur after couples split up, or as a result of online / cyberbullying. Quite often a teenager or young person will send out a naked or sexual photo to someone they trust, without really considering the implications if someone decides to break that trust. It is also being seen by teenagers as the first step in a relationship.

DID YOU KNOW?

30% of 15-year-olds have sent a naked photo of themselves at least once[39].

How do I talk to my child about revenge porn and sexting?

- Conversations about these topics should be considered in the context of general conversations about sex, children's bodies, boundaries and what is and isn't appropriate for others to touch / see. There has to be an early foundation laid to help young people understand what is and isn't acceptable and how to be in control of their body. The NSPCC has some great resources for younger children from their Let's Talk PANTS campaign, which teaches children how to stay safe (www.nspcc.org.uk).

- Make sure you talk about it with teenagers who have their own devices with cameras. If they are going to do it (because let's face it, how can you stop them?), remind them that it is less damaging to send a picture that has no identifiable features in it (no face, tattoo, birthmark, or identifiable items in the background).

- Remind them that even if their friend / partner feels like a safe and trustworthy person now, their relationship may change in the future.

- Help them understand that they have lost control of their image once they have sent it, and potentially anyone in the world could see it.

- Ask them if they would they want their friends, family, or teachers to see it, because that is what they are risking. What they are in charge of is their body and whether to send the image or not.

What should I do if my child becomes the victim of revenge porn?

- This is a highly intimate image and possibly humiliating for your child, so you will need to be very sensitive even though you are likely to feel angry and concerned. Try not to make them feel blamed, and offer them support to manage the situation.

- If your child becomes the victim of revenge porn, report it to the website or app if possible.

- As revenge porn is very serious and now illegal in the UK, some European countries and in a number of US states, you may also choose to report it to the police, so make sure you keep screenshots and records of any incidents.

- Advise your child to update their social media privacy settings, so that their content is safer and cannot be misused again.

- If appropriate, seek help from dedicated support lines such as www.revengepornhelpline.org.uk in the UK, or www.cybercivilrights.org/ in the US, who can help you and your child figure out the best course of action.

NEGATIVE IMPACT ON CHILDREN'S MENTAL HEALTH

Social media is an important space for young people and digital natives. And, as the Royal Society for Public

Health says, "it is intrinsically linked to mental health."[40] The RSPH recognise that when online, people form and build relationships, develop their unique identity, learn new things and express themselves in new ways. For that reason, social media can be really positive for mental health.

But the research on the impact of social media on children and young people's mental health is relatively new, because the social media changes rapidly and evolves on a daily basis. What we do know, though, that social media can have different effects on different people – and so it's important for you to consider how it might affect your child's mental wellbeing.

Social media can be both positive and negative for your child's mental health. Some studies report that social networking can cause exposure to harm, social isolation and depression.[41] However, research on American university students found no association between social media use and depression in older adolescents.[42]

DID YOU KNOW?

A study of secondary school pupils in the UK found that those who used social media more often and those who were more emotionally invested in social media had poorer quality sleep, lower self-esteem and higher levels of anxiety and depression.[43]

However, young people now are sharing more about themselves online than they typically would offline. They are making themselves more vulnerable, as they are also opening themselves up to a much wider audience. Certain individuals in that audience can be much less inhibited in the feedback they give, and this is called the "online disinhibition effect.

In one sense, it can be helpful for children and adolescents to widen their social circle, so that they can connect with others and feel less isolated. While there is a place for connecting with others online, it is clearly important for children and young people to develop real-world, offline relationships – particularly for those who are socially anxious.

Below are a few examples of how social media can negatively impact a child's mental health:

- Negative feedback on networking sites can decrease self-esteem and wellbeing.[44]

- Some children feel anxious about how others will see them online, making it hard to present themselves genuinely.

- Those who present a fake image of themselves online are more likely to suffer from anxiety and poor social skills.[45]

- At its worst, the internet and online gaming can become addictive and lead to a loss of interest in the real world, which has huge implications for psychological, emotional, social and academic development.

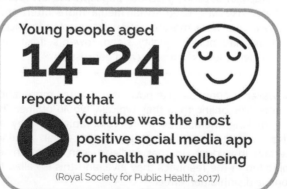

Young people aged

14-24

reported that

Youtube was the most positive social media app for health and wellbeing

(Royal Society for Public Health, 2017)

DID YOU KNOW?

Royal Society for Public Health developed a league table for the impact of social media platforms on mental health, based on 14 factors. These factors included whether the platforms made a positive or negative contribution to things such as sleep, anxiety, depression, self-expression and identity, loneliness, fear of missing out, bullying and real-world relationships.

Overall, YouTube was found to have the most positive impact. This was followed by Twitter, Facebook, Snapchat and Instagram – all of which had an overall negative impact, especially on sleep!

DAMAGING CORRELATIONS WITH BODY IMAGE ISSUES

Social media can really heavily impact upon children and young people's self-esteem, confidence and body image. The prevalence of heavily edited photos and other content reinforces the idea that children and young people are unable to live up to other people's standards, leaving them feeling inadequate and self-conscious about their looks, skills or even personalities.

How often do you post something online when you are having a difficult day, and how often do you post the good moments? How often do you look at other people's online lives and think about how good they look? The online world is giving a biased impression of real life and this can lead to unfavourable comparisons, especially amongst children and adolescents. Young people need to be reminded of this as they are developing their identity.

It's fine for them to post the good things online, but it helps to remind them that no one is perfect, and that often the content they're exposed to online is heavily edited.

The online world gives a biased impression of real life, and this can lead to children comparing themselves unfavourably, especially with their friends.

DID YOU KNOW?

In 2017, Ditch the Label's survey found that 42% of young people thought it was always okay to edit a selfie before posting it online – and therefore present a false image to the online community.[46]

Research has shown that Facebook photo activity is associated with body image disturbance in adolescent girls.[47] One study suggests that the amount of time spent posting and viewing photos positively is related to girls believing that being thin is the ideal. It also suggests links between Facebook photo activity and self-objectification, a drive towards losing weight and a lack of satisfaction with their weight.

The study did suggest, though, that engaging with photos on Facebook might be a *result* or *an expression* of girls' preoccupations with their bodies, rather than being the cause. So it's useful to keep a watchful eye on how much time your child is spending posting or looking at photographs on Facebook and pay attention to the relationship they have with their body.

Addiction to the Internet and Social Media

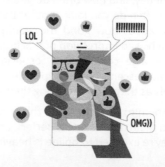

Getting lots of "likes", followers and positive comments on social media can easily become addictive! It gives you a real short-term high, so there's no wonder people love external validation and seek it out so much.

But it can have a real impact on other areas of day-to-life. Some researchers and clinicians say screens are like "digital heroin or cocaine" to children and young people, and they warn against excessive use. I've certainly seen young people who have retreated into the virtual world and struggle to spend time away from the internet! Addiction to social media can be very damaging and can have a knock-on effect in other areas of their lives, such as performance at school, relationships, and physical health.

This is a very legitimate concern. Increased use of screen time is contributing to poorer physical health as young people spend less time engaged in physical activity and more time staring at screens. As a result, they could also end up getting less sleep as they stay awake and on their phones well into the night.

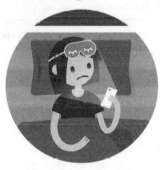

In 2015, a researcher also identified other "worrisome technology patterns," and it's easy to recognise that many of these occur due to addiction to the internet. These include:

- Abrupt change in how the child uses the internet, social media and games.

- Erratic use of the internet with lots of switching.
- Dramatic increase in electronic communication.
- Overdependence on a single online relationship.
- Avoidance of school or friends in order to stay online.
- Significant sleep impairment from online activities.
- Browser history that shows visits to suicide or self-harm sites.
- Worrisome posts or pictures on social media sites.[48]

IIn Dr Nicholas Kardaras's book, *Glow Kids*, he warns of the dangers of addiction to technology, such as "text neck" (a result of bad posture due to excessive mobile phone use), "Facebook depression" (the more friends you have online, the more likely you are to be addicted and therefore depressed, as isolation and disconnection is made worse) and gaming induced psychosis. He frames computer games as an "addicting digital drug", because rewards and stimulation cause a release of dopamine – a feel good neurotransmitter – and adrenaline, a potent and addictive combination. Some young people give up eating and sleeping to play games, and run the risk of developing ADHD and schizophrenia-type symptoms.

DID YOU KNOW?

Half of all teens in a 2016 US survey felt addicted to their device. 59% of parents felt that their kids were addicted.[49]

Research has also shown that the mere presence of a mobile phone reduces concentration[50].

CHAPTER 5

HAVE A CONVERSATION

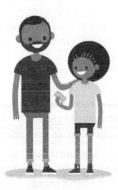

You want your child to be digitally resilient, which means that at some point you will have to talk with your child about the internet. In the same way that you help them navigate the real world, you need to support them with their online life. Help them think about what kind of person they want to be online, and that will allow you to gauge their digital savviness.

Here are some questions that you might want to consider asking when preparing to have a conversation. Don't ask them all at once, and what you ask might depend on the age of your child and their level of understanding. Pick your moment carefully, and test out whether your child is open to having a conversation at that time. The aim is to keep communication open by having gentle conversations, and not waiting until a crisis happens.

Which sites do they like to go to, what games do they like to play, and which apps do they like to use?

CONSIDER: Is there a risk of them seeing traumatising, disturbing, or age-inappropriate content on any of these platforms, or coming into contact with potentially dangerous individuals?

ACTION: Research any that you are unsure of, and explain to them why you're concerned if anything worries you. Put measures into place to help them avoid exposure to traumatising content, such as parental controls.

How do they show kindness and how do they avoid being unpleasant? Do they think it is okay to put negative comments online?

CONSIDER: Do they understand the consequences of their actions if they put negative things online or are unpleasant to social media users?

ACTION: Remind them that that even though they're behind a screen, they are still talking to real people, and their words and actions will still have a real-world effect and real-life consequences. Encourage them to think what it would be like for them to receive those comments. Help them consider how to repair any damage.

Do they think it is okay to post photos of an event if some friends weren't invited?

CONSIDER: Why are they posting these photos? Are they making sure that they are not being hurtful, or deliberately making anyone feel excluded?

ACTION: Suggest to your child that they consider the impact of posting photos of events where a friend of theirs weren't invited. Can they explain to their friends the situation so that they have an opportunity to rectify any difficulties?

Do they edit their photos and if so, why?

CONSIDER: Why do they feel the need to edit their photos? Does seeing other people's polished selfies make them feel less attractive or inadequate? How is their relationship with their body?

ACTION: Remind your child that a lot of photos and selfies online are photoshopped, airbrushed, edited or tweaked to look better than in real life – even the photos of their friends. Help them to engage in offline activities that will develop their body confidence.

What does it mean to them to get likes?

CONSIDER: How does it affect your child's self-confidence and mental wellbeing when they receive negative comments? How much of their self-worth or self-esteem is tied into likes and positive comments?

ACTION: Have a conversation with them about the importance of finding true self-confidence and affirmation from within themselves, rather than relying on the validation of others. Help them look to offline situations to develop this.

How do they deal with negative comments?

CONSIDER: Is your child able to shake off an inevitable negative comment? Do they get very upset or affected by them? How do they respond to the negative comments?

ACTION: Be sensitive about how it might feel for them. Talk together about how they manage this and see if you can develop some strategies together if necessary. Should they always respond to negative comments? Help them think about whether they are prepared to take the risk to receive negative comments by posting and whether they need to reconsider the material they are sharing.

What are they hoping to achieve when they post something?

CONSIDER: Is it important for your child to get as many "likes" or equivalent as possible? Do they have negative intentions towards others when they post?

ACTION: Discuss with them their reasons for posting a particular status, photo, comment or message. Are any of them negative? Can you help them think twice about what they are about to post, before they do so? How else can they express how they're feeling, or achieve self-confidence, without using social media first?

Are they being themselves online?

CONSIDER: Perhaps your child is pretending to be very different, or even another person altogether, while they are using the internet, gaming, or on social media. If they are doing this, what reasons could there be? Do they feel anxious or inadequate, or are they doing something dangerous or unpleasant?

ACTION: Discuss with them their reasons for posting a particular status, photo, comment or message. Are any of them negative? Can you help them think twice about what they are about to post, before they do so? How else can they express how they're feeling, or achieve self-confidence, without using social media first?

Do they share personal information and how do they keep themselves safe? Do they talk to people they don't know online? Do they understand what can happen if they share too much information and that some people lie about who they are?

CONSIDER: Depending on your child's age or digital awareness, they might not realise that sharing a lot of personal and private information can be dangerous. They also might not realise that there is a common problem with people lying about who they really are online.

ACTION: Teach your child about grooming and child sexual exploitation in an age appropriate way, explaining to them the signs and behaviours that they need to look out for. Encourage them to ask questions and raise concerns with you, or a trusted adult, if something doesn't feel right.

What does your child understand about what is safe / unsafe behaviour online?

CONSIDER: Is your child aware of the particular dangers of social media and the internet, for example online grooming or cyberbullying?

ACTION: Go back to "The Darker Side of the Internet" chapter and talk through the potential risks and dangers with them, according to what is appropriate based on their age range. Gauge their understanding and put appropriate measures in place to support them to be vigilant and sensible.

Do they know what to do if they feel unsafe or experience or witness something negative?

CONSIDER: Do they know who they can turn to when they feel unsafe online? Do they fear your judgement if they witness, or are a part of, something negative?

ACTION: Reassure them that they can come and talk to you about anything they are concerned about and identify other trusted adults who might be able to support them. You can give the contact details for organisations such Childline if you have concerns but think they are unable to talk with you.

What would they do if someone pressured them to send a picture?

CONSIDER: Do they feel confident enough, without fearing rejection, to say no when someone's pushing them for a photo they're uncomfortable sharing? Are they particularly vulnerable to peer pressure or the need to be liked? Are they aware of the potential risks of exploitation or "revenge porn" that come with sexting?

ACTION: Listen to your child empathically and stay calm, even if you don't feel it! Explain to your child the risks that come with sexting. Let them know that it is illegal for children under the age of consent (usually aged 16, but this can differ from country to country, so check the law where you live) to send out sexually explicit photos of themselves.

Do they have fear of missing out (FOMO) when they are offline? What do they think might happen if they are offline?

CONSIDER: FOMO can be a product – or a cause – of low self-esteem, low self-confidence, and / or anxiety. Your child might be having difficulties within their friendship groups, or they might not have the time or resources to do what their friends are doing.

ACTION: Empathise with their disappointment, anger, etc. about the situation. Remind them that things are very often engineered to look better than they actually are online. Reassure them that it's okay not to be involved in everything. Help them to create opportunities to spend time with friends or try out new activities.

What positives does social media give them?

CONSIDER: Social media can be a real force for good in everybody's lives. It might be a place which fosters creativity and connection for them, or provides information and learning, or helps them create social change.

ACTION: Ask them how and why social media and the internet enhances their lives in a positive way. Praise the things that are going well for them and encourage them to pursue their creativity or success in a healthy, digitally resilient way. Let them know when you notice that they have managed difficult situations well.

How have they been inspired online?

CONSIDER: Are they using certain sites or apps that inspire and encourage their creativity or involvement in activities? Perhaps they've picked up a new skill or interest because of the internet.

ACTION: Praise them for finding their creativity or motivation online. Make sure that they're using safe sources through which to explore their new ventures.

How does it help them to learn?

CONSIDER: Are they using the internet for their homework, or to pick up a new skill? Are they using verified platforms and sites that are approved by their school, educational bodies or the government?

ACTION: Praise your child for using the internet for learning. Ask them what sites or apps they're using, how they help them, and if they're credible sources. Help them find out if they're unsure. Be vigilant that they are not copying work and claiming it as their own.

Help them maintain their curiosity – how do they **know where the information comes from and how can they know if it is true?**

CONSIDER: Does your child know that something isn't necessarily true just because it's online? Do they trust information, news or rumours just because they're being circulated on big or popular apps? Maybe it hasn't occurred to them to question things more closely before sharing.

ACTION: Encourage them to question things and to be curious, especially if they plan on sharing or forwarding a post. Is there any evidence for what they're reading or seeing? Can you offer them some safe and reliable resources if they want to look something up? Encourage them to critically challenge the information they are accessing – where does it come from, who is the author, what is it based on?

Do they know that they can come and talk to you if anything worries them?

CONSIDER: Perhaps something is going on behind the scenes that they're too scared to tell you. Maybe they've done something they're not proud of. Maybe they have a big problem and they don't know who to speak to.

ACTION: Reassure them that they can come and talk to you (or, if possible, another parent, carer, professional or teacher that they trust) if they have any worries or problems. Tell them that they will not be judged or punished for being open and honest. Make sure that you are available to your child, which gives them opportunities to feel heard. Offer your undivided attention. Give them details of organisations such as Childline if you are concerned that they may not be able to share with you.

CHAPTER 6

MANAGING SOCIAL MEDIA USE AND BUILDING A PLAN

Whether we like it or not, the next generation is growing up immersed in the digital world. As parents and guardians, we have to find a way to manage this and help our children navigate the virtual world as safely and happily as possible.

There is no one central place for all recommendations, but the idea of this chapter is to help you think about how you would like to manage your family's use of the internet and social media.

Research shows that more and more parents are taking steps to monitor and manage their child's internet use, including using parental controls and talking to children about how to use it safely. And there's no doubt about it – prevention is better than cure!

It's important to recognise that in today's digital world, social media is important to young people and it's likely to play a big part in everyone's day-to-day lives.

The world offline should be as, if not more, interesting than the online world, and face-to-face communication should be enjoyable! However, we all know that people – children and young people especially – spend a lot of their spare time interacting with people online, and so it's best to promote your child's online resilience in the same way that you help them learn how to get along in the real world

– how to form relationships with others, how to problem solve and how make sense of information given to them.

How strict should I be when setting rules?

Think about your parenting style and how it relates to how you manage technology as a family. Gold (2015) uses the below model to show how different parenting styles result in different types of control over family internet use.

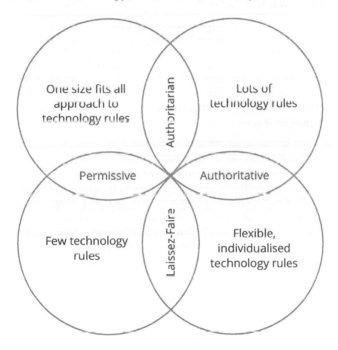

She suggests that "authoritative parents" are best positioned to promote online resilience. This parenting style recognises that children have individual needs, and therefore a flexible approach is needed. Authoritative parents recognise the need for a number of technology rules in the household, but they also recognise that those rules need to be *flexible* where needed and individualised to the family member.

Therefore, you need to understand your family and your child and think about how you will help them manage social media depending on their age, level of understanding, interests, how able they are to manage themselves safely online, and how easily they can come away from screens.

BUILDING A PLAN

The American Association for Paediatrics (AAP) recommends that all families create a technology plan and / or a contract for their home. That way, parents can feel reassured that the internet and social media is being used safely and sensibly in their home, with everyone agreeing to play their part.

But before doing this, the first thing to consider is your own use of social media. Ask yourself some questions and figure out what an ideal scenario is for your family based on honest answers. What are you happy or unhappy with? What behaviours and habits do you have with social media and the internet that you wouldn't like them to pick up themselves? What positive social media habits would you like to demonstrate to them? Remember, children learn about internet usage from you before they even begin to use it, and teenagers and adolescents may look to you as an example or as a justification for their own habits.

Here are some questions for you to consider, with space to answer. You can do this on a separate piece of paper if you wish.

- **How often do I use social media?**

- **What device(s) do I use?**

- **When do I use it? When my child(ren) are present? At meal times? Before bed? In bed? During conversations?**

- **Do I have time without my device?**

- **Do I sleep with my device(s)?**

_____

_____

_____

- **What might I be teaching my child about social media use?**

_____

_____

- **Which of my bad habits would I like them not to pick up and why?**

_____

_____

_____

- **Which of my positive habits would I like them to take on?**

_____

_____

_____

- **Do I know what to do if someone is behaving inappropriately online?**

_____

_____

_____

- **Do I understand the privacy settings of the social media I use?**

_____

_____

_____

- **Is my personal information safe?**

_____

_____

_____

_____

- **Can other people view pictures that I post of my child?**

_____

_____

_____

- **Do I seek permission from other parents before posting pictures online?**

_____

_____

_____

- **How often are they on social media and how much time do they spend online?**

_____

_____

_____

- **What device(s) do they use?**

_____

_____

_____

_____

- **Where do they use their device(s)?**

_____

_____

_____

- **How well supervised are they when online?**

- **How are they spending their time online? (Do they use it for social media, online gaming, watching TV / films / vlogs, or using it for homework?)**

- **What are their ages and stages and what would you like them to be doing while offline?**

- **At this stage, how digitally resilient is your child? What, if anything, do they understand about the risks?**

- **How do they keep themselves safe, and how do they manage when they experience negative feedback?**

  _____

  _____

- **What kind of online identity do they have? How do they interact with others online?**

  _____

  _____

  _____

  _____

  _____

- **Do they have respect and empathy for others?**

  _____

  _____

  _____

  _____

  _____

  _____

- **Are they presenting a genuine image of themselves without giving too much personal information away?**

  _____

  _____

- **Who would they talk to If they were struggling with something online?**

  _____

  _____

  _____

- **Do they know what is / isn't okay to download?**

  _____

  _____

  _____

  _____

- **Which of my positive habits would I like them to take on?**

  _____

  _____

  _____

  _____

YOUR FAMILY'S RULES

Now that you have identified what's important to you and your family and how you want your child to stay safe, think about the rules that you would like to set within your household and how you will go about exploring them, agreeing them with your partner or other carers, and sharing them with your child.

You will need to balance the needs of children of different ages, each of whom will need different rules and consequences. You will need to communicate this need effectively with them.

Here are some areas to consider when putting together a plan:

TIMING AND LOCATION

It's best to consider how much time you believe your child should be allowed to spend online. There is no right or wrong answer for this, but it's important that you have an idea of what you want before building it into a plan.

Do you want to have a digital curfew? What time should your child switch off for the night? You might decide that there should be no screen time at least an hour, or more or less, before bedtime. If you factor a curfew into your plan, it's a good idea to give them reminders as the time approaches, so that they don't lose track of time. You might also advise or instruct your child to put their screens on night mode in the evenings.

Where and when are you happy for your child to go online? Will you decide that there can be no phones at the table and / or no internet use before homework? Can they use their device(s) in the bedroom, in the living room, when travelling in the car? Will you allow your child to sleep with their device?

Do you want to have family time offline? If so, for how long (for example, a minimum of 30 minutes a day)? How will you all spend this time together?

CONTENT

What social media apps and websites will you allow your child to use? How will you monitor this? Are there certain sites that you don't want them view? Are they posting content that you believe they should seek permission from friends or family to use?

SAFETY AND ONLINE CONDUCT

Do you want to establish agreements about what is and isn't acceptable to share on social media? What safeguards are you comfortable putting into place? Will you agree that your child should let you follow them online, and would you like to set up parental controls?

Would you like to set up rules for conduct and what is forbidden, for example sharing personal information, cyberbullying, setting up fake accounts, sexting, copying others' work, buying / selling online?

Will you follow our child on social media sites such as Facebook? How will you agree whether it is okay to comment or like their posts?

Will you discuss with your child the importance of thinking twice before they share content?

BUILDING YOUR PLAN

Family internet and social media plans can take any shape or format. Basically, they should be a written form of the agreements that you and your family make regarding social media.

You can set out your plan as a simple list of family rules which acts as a contract, and then get each family member to sign it to say they agree and commit to following them.

You could also set it out in a table, with different rules under different family members' names.

If you are a teacher, you could also build a plan or list of rules that clearly sets out the boundaries for social media use within your classroom.

CONSEQUENCES

Now is the time to think about what will happen if the rules are broken. Perhaps you can discuss possible consequences with someone else, e.g. your partner, before building them into your plan and letting your child know what these are. It's important that the adults are on the same page and have a level of agreement about consequences.

It's better to think about what options you have before something happens. It's also okay to take some time to think about what should happen next. After all, that's better than impulsively blurting out something that's over the top, hard to enforce and likely to build resentment!

You'll want to keep lines of communication open, and extreme punishments can cause ill feeling within families and stop this happening.

What options do you have for consequences of broken rules?

Examples include:

- Removal of a device for a period of time (an hour, a day, two days).

- Turning off the wifi / internet (think about the impact on others).

- Removal of a privilege.

- Doing something to earn a device back, such as a household chore.

Make the punishment / consequences proportionate and something that will teach them a valuable lesson. For example:

- Having your child write an apology to someone for making negative comments.

- Ask them to research the risks of disclosing personal information and read them out to you – this helps them with learning digital resilience!

- Talk to them and help them with their homework if they copy from the internet.

HERE ARE SOME TIPS FOR DEVELOPING YOUR PLAN:

- Set clear boundaries for internet use as soon as possible and be consistent.

- Make sure everyone completely understands the rules in the plan, and make sure there is no ambiguity.

- Talk to your child and ask them if they have any concerns about the rules and why.

- Print out your plan / list of rules / social media agreement and display it somewhere in your house where everyone can see it.

- Review your agreement regularly and make changes as needed.

If you would like a downloadable template for a contract or social media plan, please visit the Social Media and Mental Health books page on www.triggerpublishing.com

**If you found this book interesting ...
why not read this next?**

Social Media and Mental Health

Handbook for Teens :)

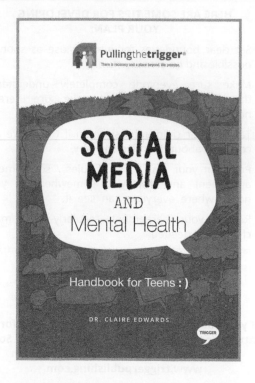

Social Media and Mental Health Handbook for Teens :) is the
perfect guide for teenagers on how to navigate the rocky
waters of the online world.

If you found this book interesting ...
why not read this next?

You can get our Social Media and Mental Health Handbooks as a two-book bundle.

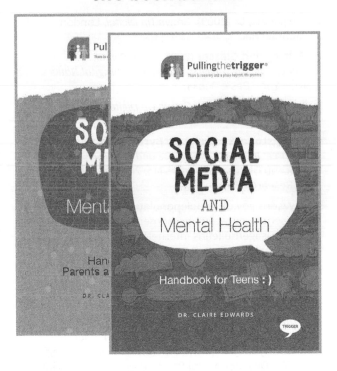

Our Social Media and Mental Health Handbooks are invaluable in helping teenagers and their guardians to stay safe online.

REFERENCES

1   **Taspscott, D.** (2009). *Grown Up Digital.* London: McGraw Hill.

2   **Palfrey and Glasser** (2008). *Born Digital: Understanding the First Generation of Digital Natives.* New York: Basic Books.

3   **Taspscott, D.** (2009). *Grown Up Digital.* London: McGraw Hill.

4   **Livingstone, S., Carr, J., & Byrne, J.** (2016). *One in Three: Internet Governance and Children's Rights.* Inocenti Discussion Papers No. 2016-01. UNICEF Office of Research. Florence.

5   www.ons.gov.uk peoplepopulationandcommunity/ householdcharacteristicshomeinternetandsocial mediausage/bulletins internetaccesshouseholdsand individuals/2016

6   **Siegel, D. & Payne Bryson, T.** (2012). *The Whole Brain Child.* London: Robinson.

7   **Ferguson, C. J., & Donnellan, M. B.** (2013, July 15). *Is the Association Between Children's Baby Video Viewing and Poor Language Development Robust? A Reanalysis of Zimmerman, Christakis, and Meltzoff* (2007). Developmental Psychology (Advance online publication). DOI: 10.1037/a0033628

8   **Gold, J.** (2015). *Screen Smart Parenting: How to Find Balance and Benefit in Your Child's Use of Social Media, Apps and Digital Devices,* by J. Gold, Child

& Family Behavior Therapy, 37:2, 163-173. DOI: 10.1080/07317107.2015.1035994

9 **Summers, P., DeSollar-Hale, A., Ibrahim-Leathers, H.** (2013). *Toddlers on Technology*. AuthorHouse.

10 **Ofcom.** (2017). *Children and Parents: Media Use and Attitudes Report.*

11 **Ofcom.** (2016, 2017). *Children and Parents: Media Use and Attitudes Report.*

12 Ofcom, 2016 and 2017. *Children and Parents: Media Use and Attitudes Report*

13 **Livingstone, S.** (2017). EU Kids Online. In: *Hobbs, Renee, (ed.) The International Encyclopedia of Media Literacy.* Wiley-Blackwell, Oxford, UK. (In Press)

14 **Ofcom.** (2016, 2017). *Children and Parents: Media Use and Attitudes Report.*

15 **Ofcom.** (2016). Children and Parents: *Media Use and Attitudes Report.*

16 **Ofcom.** (2016). Children and Parents: *Media Use and Attitudes Report.*

17 **Ofcom.** (2016). *Children and Parents: Media Use and Attitudes Report.*

18 **Ofcom.** (2016). *Children and Parents: Media Use and Attitudes Report.*

19 **Ofcom.** (2016). *Children and Parents: Media Use and Atitudes Report.*

20 www.bbc.co.uk/news/business-40424769, accessed 3rd July 2017

21 **Children's Commissioner,** Jan 2017. *Growing Up Digital: A Report of the Growing Up Digital Taskforce.* London, 2017.

22 https://horizon-magazine.eu/article/least-5-young-people-suffer-symptoms-social-media-addiction_en.html [accessed 01/02/18]

23 www.ccam-ascor.nl/images/2015_Lemmens_
Valkenburg_Gentile_InternetGamingDisorderScale-
PsychologicalAssessment2015.pdf [accessed 01/02/18]

24 www.ccam-ascor.nl/images/2015_Lemmens_
Valkenburg_Gentile_InternetGamingDisorderScale-
PsychologicalAssessment2015.pdf [accessed 01/02/18]

25 www.ccam-ascor.nl/images/2015_Lemmens_
Valkenburg_Gentile_InternetGamingDisorderScale-
PsychologicalAssessment2015.pdf [accessed 01/02/18]

26 **Allen, K., Ryan, T., Gray, D., McInerney, D., &
Waters, L.** (2014). *Social Media Use and Social
Connectedness in Adolescents: The Positives and the
Potential Pitfalls.* The Australian Educational and
Developmental Psychologist, 31(1), 18-31. DOI:10.1017/
edp.2014.2

27 **Valkenburg, P. M., Peter, J. & Schouten, A. P.** (2006).
*Friend networking sites and their relationship
to adolescents' well-being and social self-esteem.*
CyberPsychology & Behavior, 9(5), 584-590

28 **Best, P., Manktelow, R. & Taylor, B.J.** (2014).
*Online Communication, Social Networking and Adolescent
Wellbeing: A Systemic Narrative Review.* Children and
Youth Services Review, 41, 27-36.

29 **Ofcom.** (2017). *Children and Parents: Media Use and
Attitudes Report*

30 www.stopspeaksupport.com/about [accessed 25.01.18]

31 www.change.org/p/app-store-google-play-ban-apps-
like-sarahah-where-my-daughter-was-told-to- kill-
herself www.change.org/p/google-inc-help-stop-
anonymous-apps-like-yik-yak-after-school-and-slam-
high-by-changing-apple-and-google-s-app-rules

32 www.ditchthelabel.org/research-papers/the-annual-
bullying-survey-2017/ accessed 24.01.18

33 www.getcybersafe.gc.ca/cnt/cbrbllng/prnts/chld-bng-
cbrblld-en.aspx

34 www.internetmatters.org/parental-controls/

35 **Przybblski, A., Murayama, K., DeHaan, C., & Gladwell, V.** (2013). Motivational, Emotional and Behavioural Correlates of Fear of Missing Out. *Computers in Human Behaviour, 29*, 1841–1848.

36 **Georgia M. Winters & Elizabeth L. Jeglic.** (2017) Stages of Sexual Grooming: Recognizing Potentially Predatory Behaviors of Child Molesters, Deviant Behavior, 38:6, 724-733, DOI:10.1080/01639625.2016.1197656

37 www.nspcc.org.uk [accessed 27.01.18]

38 **Ofcom.** (2016). *Children and Parents: Media Use and Attitudes Report*

39 www.ditchthelabel.org/research-papers/the-wireless-report/

40 **#StatusofMind:** Social media and young people's mental health www.rsph.org.uk/uploads/assets/uploaded/62be270a-a55f-4719-ad668c2ec7a74c2a.pdf [accessed 01.02.18]

41 **Valkenburg, P.M., Peter, J. & Schouten, A.P.** (2006). Friend networking sites and their relationship to adolescents; well-being and social self-esteem. *Cyberpsychology & Behavior, 9*(5), 584-590.

42 **Jelenchick, Eickhoff & Moreno** (2012). "Facebook Depression?" Social Networking Site Use and Depression in Older Adolescents. *Journal of Adolescent Health, 7*, 128-30.

43 **Woods, H.C. and Scott, H.** (2016). #Sleepyteens: social media use in adolescence is associated with poor sleep quality, anxiety, depression and low seld-esteem. *Journal of Adolescence, 51*, 41-49.

44 **Valkenburg, P.M., Peter, J. & Schouten, A.P.** (2006). Friend networking sites and their relationship to adolescents; well-being and social self-esteem. *CyberPsychology & Behavior, 9*(5), 584-590.

45 Harman, J.P., Hansen, C.E., Cochran, M.E. & Lindsey, C.R. (2005). Liar, Liar: Internet faking but not frequency of use affects social skills, self-esteem, social anxiety and aggression. *CyberPsychology and Behavior, 8*(1), 1-6.

46 www.ditchthelabel.org/wp-content/uploads/2017/07/The-Annual-Bullying-Survey-2017-1.pdf

47 Meier, E.P.,& Gray, J. (2014). Facebook Photo activity associated with body image disturbance in adolescent girls. *Cyberpsychology, Behavior and Social Networking, 17*(4), 199-206.

48 Gold, J. (2015). *Screen-Smart Parenting: How to Find Balance and Benefit in Your Child's Use of Social Media, Apps, and Digital Devices.* The Guildford Press: London

49 www.commonsensemedia.org/about-us/news/press-releases/new-report-finds-teens-feel-addicted-to-their-phones-causing-tension-at

50 Thornton, B., Faires, A., Robbins, M., & Rollins, E. (2014). The Mere Presence of a Cell Phone May Be Distracting: Implications for Attention and Task Performance. *Social Psychology, 45*(6), 479-488.

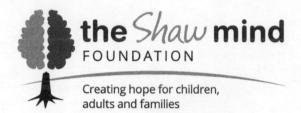

the *Shaw* mind
FOUNDATION

Creating hope for children,
adults and families

Sign up to our charity, The Shaw Mind Foundation

www.shawmindfoundation.org

and keep in touch with us; we would love to hear
from you.

*Our goal is to make help and support available for every
single person in society, from all walks of life.
We will never stop offering hope. These are our promises.*